STOP OVERTHINKING

PART 1

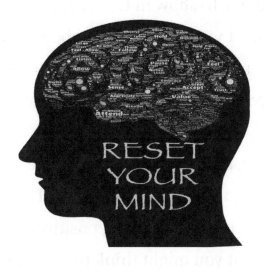

Mindfulness, Meditation, and Positive Thinking

The ability I 'd like to show in this chapter is all about being conscious. I would like to talk about three forms of awareness, although they are all closely related and are part of each other. I want to mention all three mostly because they are often interchangeable, and if you don't recognize one, I'm sure you're going to hear about another. They are mindful, meditating and thinking positively.

Now, it's true that you might think positive thinking isn't the same as mindfulness and meditation, but I think positive thinking is a form of meditation in many ways, and I'm going to explain it in a little bit. First, let's define a little clearer the mindfulness.

Mindfulness

When I say the word "mindfulness," many people often think of the phrase "paying attention" automatically. If that's what you thought about, you 're not wrong! Paying attention to what you are doing, your environment, and how you feel is an important part of your mindfulness practice. But it goes deeper than just paying attention, and it's harder than it sounds for most people.

Mindfulness is a practice of being present over the course of your life, not just for a minute or two, but throughout the day, each day. The goal is to maintain constant awareness, although we all accept that we are not computers or robots, and there will be times when we lose focus or our minds are filled with other emotions and feelings that take us away in response to events in life. A religious mindset can draw a parallel. Followers in the Christian mindset accept that they are human and make mistakes, while at the same time doing their best every day to maintain a sinless, just, and faithful existence. Just because we know we 're going to be making mistakes; that doesn't mean we 're not trying. And that is why our efforts are well worth the long-term effects emotionally, spiritually, physically and emotionally. Let's look at what awareness has to offer us and then learn how to integrate the practice into your own life.

Consider how you feel after banishing a wasteful or hurtful thinking effectively and replacing it with a different, optimistic one. You feel good, doesn't it? And it also gives you a sense of clarity, just like a big mess from your mind's floor has just been cleansed. When we learn to practice mindfulness, the same thing happens. There is a bonus just with carefulness. Practicing mindfulness consistently leads to a feeling of potential, hope and a fresh pair of eyes looking forward. With a clear mind, you move forward and you take stock of every second that passes you by. So, I don't talk about looking forward to the next day or weekend or month when I'm talking about a feeling of potential and looking forward. I'm talking about moving forward, step-by-step, minute-by-minute, feeling and seeing everything around you and feeling as it goes through every moment. There's a sense of peace and fulfillment that comes when you're getting rid of the feelings that don't mean a difference to you at the time. And thank you, your face.

Thank your heart and soul. There's so much to love for here right now, to be thankful. Mindfulness is all about getting such near quarters into your mind, a small-scale way of living, and the entire world opens up to you in the process.

So, how do you start your mindfulness practice? Well, the biggest task here will be to upgrade focus skills. But the news is good. If you were able to practice the technique of interruption and replace your negative thoughts and emotions with positive ones, then you have already done a great deal to cultivate this skill. Focus comes from the mental effort of sharpening your thinking and scaling it down to a single task without allowing your mind to wander around the place to things that don't help you accomplish that. You do not want to fall into the trap of trying so hard as to make this exercise a chore and a source of worry for you, as I've discussed before.

Anyone new to mindfulness and first introduced will move forward and improve at a different pace because we are unique human beings. And this is perfectly fine. As with everything else in this book, taking small steps at a time is the key.

A good exercise in mindfulness practice is simply going outside and experiencing nature. Go to a generally quiet area of a park and take a seat at a bench or picnic table. Take some deep breaths, and calm your mind. To accomplish this give yourself a minute or two. Listen to the noises that are going on around you, the dogs barking or the breeze rushing through the trees when you start concentrating your attention. Feel the wind on your skin, or the sun's fire beating down on you. Feel like the body is in vacuum.

Make sure you have a good seating spot. €Lose your eyes as you start out. Then open your eyes slowly as you start to appreciate and focus only on what's around you. Look around and take in what you see without thinking about them. Again, that may not come with practice naturally, but gradually. Enjoy the beauty that is around you whatever you see. You can do the same exercise in your own backyard or neighborhood, if you don't have a nice park to go to. Hear the birds or the children running down the lane. Try to focus only on sensations without forming thoughts or allowing your mind to wander around. As you spend time practicing awareness for just a few minutes each day, you will begin to notice that the more you practice, the easier it becomes.

Meditation

A discussion of awareness naturally follows into a meditation discussion because they are closely related. For me, though they suggest separate activities, they are part of each other.

For many people, meditation translates into practicing mindfulness every day. To some, meditation means a fixed period of time every day or week that is used by a single school of thought or philosophy for formal meditation practice. Zen Buddhism, for example, I'm going to mention a few different meditation styles, but I'm going to talk about Zen in particular because it's the form I'm most familiar with.

The same exercises that you have learned in nature can extend to a meditation activity. Since most people associate meditation with the image of sitting in a quiet room with your eyes closed, let 's look at how you can start practicing meditation in your own home with a few simple steps to follow.

Find a relaxed position, based on your physical capacity, where you can sit fairly straight with the back. You should relax your arms at your sides and not strain your neck. If you are interested in this, a simple Google search will go through the more formal sitting structure, but we'll take a casual approach to the physical technique for now and focus more on what's going on inside your mind.

When we talked about mindfulness, we talked about sensing the world around you and just focusing on what's happening to you right now.

Meditation is similar, except that in the Zen meditation practice, the aim is not to regulate one 's thoughts, but rather to avoid clinging to particular thoughts while they enter and leave the mind. The central emphasis is still to concentrate on the moment, but Zen 's theory is not to restrain the mind but instead to free the mind and let it remain flexible while referring to the current reality regularly.

To explain this, have you ever found yourself or a friend found you spacing out, looking blankly in front of you, as your mind drifts and starts to have a conversation with itself over what you said yesterday or what that may have been humiliating for years? The process of thinking has taken you out of the present altogether, and now you are lost in a replay of moments that have already happened, things that can not be changed. But still, you dwell as mistakes on those moments and worry about what people think about you, while they probably don't even remember those insignificant events in reality. Comfortable sound? We 're just doing the same. The ultimate goal in meditation is to avoid those sticky thoughts that try their best to take us out of the present and into the past or the future — spaces that can't be changed or we can't foresee. In an effort to predict and make sense of our lives, the brain likes to know things and to form patterns. But we can get wrapped up in this to the point where we are missing life as it happens in the present.

Zen is all about acknowledging the wandering nature of the mind but also accepting the core principle of impermanence, that is, it changes everything, even the thoughts in your mind. In an impermanent universe, focusing on a single thought or feeling or emotion is pointless and meaningless, and can keep you only at a standstill. This does not yet make complete sense, and if you need to continue with the absolute fundamentals, go back to the term we mentioned at the beginning of this essay.

Just "look around," feel yourself in space, listen, appreciate. That's all you need to focus on in order to get started. You will soon form a new addiction to the positivity that awareness offers, as with all these positive habits. Meditation will follow naturally after this point.

As I mentioned earlier, meditation can take many forms and you shouldn't feel there's one way to meditate. Via dancing to music, many practice mindfulness and meditation, called dance meditation. Other people, including Zen Buddhist monks, practice "walking meditation." Movements often help to regulate and soothe the mind as we introduce movement patterns that flow just as our thoughts flow free. Whatever your style and preference, all you need to do is remember why you practice first and there is no "doing it wrong."

Positive Thinking

Good thinking ties right in with the methodology of thought where we replaced negative ideas and added constructive ones. But with positive thinking, the idea is first to cultivate the positive thoughts, rather than wait and use them as a reaction to negative thoughts. This is another practice which will look different from one person to another. It should also not be an intimidating idea that would stop you from trying it out.

Positive thinking simply means that you practice waking up and thinking of each day as a fresh, new, unpredictable day, rather than dreading what you think you know will happen. No one knows the future, because even though your life appears to be fairly set in stone, when you're in the habit of dreading something every day in conjunction with work (which I think you've already addressed!), otherwise you close yourself to witnessing new events or stuff that will make you content. You may know an example of what I'm talking about. Think of Mr. Scrooge from the classic Christmas story, "A Christmas Carol." It's Christmas Eve and there are kids smiling and playing in the snow, people shopping and exchanging Christmas cards, and joyfully chatting with strangers. Yet then there's Mr. Scrooge trudging for his office in the snow, already realizing that Christmas is a miserable time because there's no joy to be had in it — only money loss. Because he's already determined he won't enjoy Christmas, he can't open his heart to the joy that happens all around him.

Similarly, we become blind to the events that would offer joy and surprise and happiness when we wake up and dread what will happen that day.

Were you aware that when you're upset or unhappy, people receive subtle signals not to engage with you or talk to you? Think of all the fun spontaneous conversations you've had in the workplace when you arrive in a good mood, positive and open to anything that the day will throw at you. Let this thought be a motivation for you every day, at the start of the day, to try to cultivate positive thinking.

Cultural Backing for the Effects of Positive Thinking

You may or may not remember the "law of attraction" phenomenon, as it was popularized through releases such as The Secret. Many claim that when you practice, regularly optimistic thinking really helps to trigger positive experiences and outcomes in your life. You've always heard the saying, "When you set your mind to it, you can do something." That's what good thinking is all about, and the law of attraction.

As you practice this skill, it may help journalising about your experience. Talk of a reason for your future. Perhaps it's a dream you've had for years and years or maybe it's something you've only been talking about today. Write down your goal in your journal and write down a little bit about what it might look like for you to achieve that goal. You may see yourself at a big party with a family and friends as you celebrate a promotion, or you have set aside time for a family holiday in the Bahamas. Perhaps you're visualizing that you've lost 30 pounds in that new bathing suit that you've had your eye on for a long time. Whatever the target, the aim here is to write down as much detail as you can think about the encounter. Make it truly real in your mind and then write down what you see.

Next, you'll want to write down the moves towards the target on the roadmap. Positive thought is a strong tool, but you'll still need to put in the time to make your target a reality. What should you do between now and next year to help you attain your promotion? What strategy will you have to adopt to lose weight successfully and in a way that you can sustain?

If you watch movie awards shows, you may be familiar with the speech that many of the winners are giving in which they attest to years of visualizing and thinking about their dreams before they actually accomplish what they wanted.

If you let yourself be depressed and convince yourself that you can never achieve anything, then you definitely won't. Practicing constructive thoughts would inevitably get you closer and closer to your goals, as you are knowingly and subconsciously encouraging yourself to be prepared for the chances that you will potentially skip in a pessimistic attitude. Much like Scrooge and his indifference to happiness, you can wrap yourself in misery so closely that you don't see a chance right in front of you.

Practice positive thinking and awareness each and every day in small steps, and it will soon become easy and natural to continue. The happiness and liberation that comes with this kind of activity is something that the mind and body and soul will start longing for. Much as when you workout and your body thanks you for all the positive endorphin emotions and a sense of success, the mind and body will reward you for the future for optimistic thoughts, and it will become impossible to fight the lure of positivity.

Do not just take my word for it. If you are working hard to cultivate and maintain these positive changes in your life, I 'm positive that as they witness the changes happening, you'll hear about it from those closest to you. It can even motivate them to learn more about mindfulness, meditation, and positive thinking so as to also make these practices an important part of their lives.

PART 2

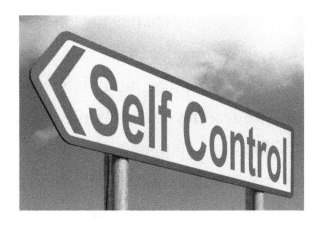

Overthinking: Putting a STOP

Accept Not Being in Control

I am convinced that what happens to me is 10 percent of life and 90 percent of how I react to it." -Charles R. Swindling

Mr Swindoll sounds very enlightened, but what does that assertion mean? You can't manage anything about your life, so it can't change the amount of curiosity, fear, or reconsider the circumstance. Relinquishing control can be intimidating for an overthinker's controlling nature. While you can't control anything that's happening in your life, you can only control your reaction to it. Hold that in mind. Live by the words. Repeat them to yourself when necessary. A person who controls their external responses is in charge of their lives. You can choose for yourself how to interpret and respond to any situation. This chapter will give examples of situations where you might find yourself ruminating about what you have done wrong to cause the perceived problem and offer alternative thinking processes to end the cycle of destructive thinking. Take a minute to enumerate the triggers list. Triggers are situations where you often find yourself, rather than acting, worrying, overanalyzing or procrastinating. Examples of common triggers include:

-Too much time alone. For negative thoughts too much free time can serve as an amusement park.

- Sleep deprived. You may find yourself making gross over-generalizations when you've not been sleeping well.

- Doing poorly. Eating a diet that allows nutritional deficiencies has been associated with reduced awareness, and increased stress and anxiety.

Recognizing the causes helps you recognise and take steps to avoid the opportunity for harmful behaviour. Agree that you can't control every single moment of your day, but you can only control how you react. Take control of your emotions, and let go of your need to control all else.

Will you take an active decision to let go of frustration, worry, or anger? Or are you going to lose sleep, harm relationships, and carry on a life of overthinking? Your choice and yours alone. Let's apply that concept to situations in the real world.

SITUATION 1: TRAFFIC

Even the quietest of people can be prone to losing their cool in a rush hour. See it: Commute the Monday morning. You 're well-rested, your morning went smoothly, and so will the rest of your day. You have created an environment in which actionable success is welcome. Anything can ruin this day with a plan! Your favorite song is on the radio, and the coffee is at a perfect temperature when a sports car gets out of nowhere and sweeps into your lane, cutting you off effectively. Quick braking stops an crash so you're a mess now. Perfect coffee now lies all over your previously flawless outfit. This is the moment when you have to make a choice. Will you spend the day dwelling on or decide to move past this incident? Know nobody can make you feel bad. Your decision taking is the result of how you want to react.

Reaction 1: Under your breath, Mother rude comments for the rest of the drive becoming angrier with the offender. Claim to anyone in the office who listens to the event, showing the coffee stains like a battle wound in civil war. Spend the day busy because about all the things a poor driver might or could have done to stop being cut off. Your list for the day wasn't finished at the end of the day and now you have to drive home, hoping that someone isn't cutting you off again. Your partner at home makes the mistake of asking how your day went and you're still upset by the jerk that cut you off, stained your clothes, caused you not to get your work done for the day, and you're surprised that you've made it home without another traffic incident, etc. "Looks like everyone has a Monday event," Office Space said best.

Reaction 2: Sense your frustration for a moment. Then realize that you could have done nothing to control the situation, opt to let it go. Think of any reason to be grateful, you 're actually wearing your coffee, but otherwise unscathed, choosing to move on. Go on business as usual, complete your daily task list and go home feeling accomplished. You can honestly reply when your partner asks about your day that you have had a positive and productive day.

SITUATION 2: INTERVIEW TO JOB

You are applying for a great job and are enthusiastic about an interview when you contact them. This is the point where the pain continues with an overthinker. With rapid speed, unwelcome thoughts start to pop up in your head. "I'm not even qualified to work remotely. What was it that I felt to go there? What if I turn myself into a fool? What do I wear? "And so forth. You have well thought out the answers for every question during the interview. So skepticism starts to crawl in as you step into the parking lot. Are you going to question your every word until you regret even applying for the job or accept that whatever happens now is out of your control?

Reaction 1: Spend hours rethinking each reply. What did you mean to wear those socks? The interviewer thinks you 're probably a fraud. Instead, what do you say? During one of your replies, the interviewer made a face. Don't bother to send a thank you note, because they won't consider you anyway for the position. Lose sleep thinking and rethink every detail of the interview and how you got it messed up. When your spouse asks about the interview, provide them with a list of every reason that you shouldn't have applied first.

Reaction 2: Take the knowledge out of the interview that you had very good answers to the questions, and ask appropriate questions about the position. Send the interviewer a brief note to thank them for their time, and move on. Understand that at this stage the result is outside of your power.

Situation 3: A (Real or Imagined) Conflict

At times, any relationship experiences a difference. Romantic, platonic, and personal partnerships are subject from time to time to varying views. Your supervisor is not in agreement with your idea about a proposal. You may not be talking to a friend and you are not sure why. When you asked for gold, your spouse bought some red wine. Will you cling to the anger/disappointment or will you get up above? Again it's your choice.

Reaction 1: Assume that your boss thinks all your ideas are undignified. Offer none when asked for input in future meetings, for fear of further rejection. Spend time reflecting about every previous interaction, and ask if you should have done better to make your manager more like you. Never call your friend to clear up the issue, but spend hours playing on an internal, endless loop, the last conversation you had with him. To think over and again what you have done wrong without even realizing their absence has nothing to do with you. Brood over dinner, because your seafood dish was not paired well with the wine. Dream all night about the bottle, and how much better it should have been. Wonder how the conversation with your spouse could have changed to prevent this mistake from happening.

Reaction 2: Continue with the initial project design. You put forward the idea, it's been rejected, you move on. Nothing ventured as they say, nothing gained. Choose not to become personally offended or allocate unwarranted concern to the issue. When asked for input, offer ideas and recognize that even if they don't always agree, your boss probably values your opinion. Check with your mate. Have a rational discussion if you have upset them and then move on with the knowledge that the conflict has been resolved. If their silence had nothing to do with you, then accept and move on with this truth. Thank you for telling your friend of the wine and acknowledging that it was a error rather than a clear result of what you might have done differently. Move step beyond the dispute. The first mentioned responses are packed with thoughts which are considered perceptual hallucinations. Cognitive distortions are, inaccurate evaluations that promote negative thinking or feelings. The good thing is, you don't need to resort to the disappointment. A further alternative is cognitive rehabilitation, as emulated by the second reactions.

Challenging your assumptions and exploring different meanings is a way to consciously avoid running over your mind with pessimistic feelings.

In the traffic situation, the prevalent types of distortions represented are catastrophization and blaming. Catastrophizing attributes more meaning to an event than it merits while blaming is the thought that somebody has made you feel a certain way. One act of inconsiderate conduct from another is the explanation behind your lack of success, bad thoughts and an awkward discussion over dinner when they made you feel frustrated all day long.

Instead, restructure your thinking to recognize that your reaction to the one event can affect the rest of the day drastically. Accept the other driver made an error and leave it at that. Stop for a new cup of coffee, be thankful that the coffee didn't cause burns and then turn back on your favorite song. Start up where you left off to get on with the day with the list of things to do.

Filtering and jumping to conclusions in the job interview situation, are the forms of cognitive distortions. Filtering concentrates small negative information while ignoring all positive aspects of the incident. The process of filtering leads you to leap to the conclusion that you did not serve

You're well and won't be picked as a consequence of the work. Your negative assumption is accepted as fact. Restructured thinking helps you to be thankful for the opportunities you have had to reflect yourself to the best of your abilities and wait quietly to know the outcome. What's done is done and the outcomes are beyond your control.

The three scenarios of disagreement allow for any form of cognitive distortion. Filtering until only a fraction of your relationship is recognized, jumping to the conclusion that your boss is not your friend anymore. Blaming your boss, friend, and spouse for making yourself feel negative. Catastrophizing the result of the wine mix up until convinced that the perfect dinner was completely ruined. Instead, restructure your thinking to consider that your boss thought you had a great idea but his boss gave them strict instructions. Give them when asked for potential suggestions, with the expectation that they would not inquire if they did not want the advice. Remember consciously your mate doesn't ignore you. Maybe, she's got a big workload or she doesn't feel good lately. What other reasons could your spouse have had for buying the wrong wine? He may have had a hard day at work and was at the shop concerned. Maybe he knows that your usual go-to is a red one, and he thought by choosing your favorite type he was doing a nice thing.

At the end of the day, fully accepting that you are not in control of the world around you can save you from hours of anger , frustration, sadness, worry, self-doubt and destructive overthinking resulting from those feelings. There is no one who can make you feel that way. Your feelings are one of the few things you absolutely have control over. Embrace the fact that you have control of the sensations. In less than optimal conditions allow a decision to feel healthy. Check again at the Trigger Situations list. Practice telling yourself that in response to any event you can only control your thoughts and actions, and that you can not control the event itself. When you continue to think about things outside of your influence, echo Mr. Charles R. Swindoll's words, "Life is 10 percent what's happening to me and 90 percent how I'm reacting to it."

Face Your Fear

Fear often constitutes the root of overthinking and procrastination. Everyone is experiencing fear, but you can choose to face and take steps to overcome irrational fear. Eliminating your fears ensures that you identify the causes. Is too many media inspiring bad feelings towards the world and your place within it? Do you find that when shopping you compare yourself to the models or mannequins? Are you loving swimming but avoiding the pool out of fear that people will think you 're too skinny or not enough? Were you scared to ask the young guy at work to go and have a drink because he thinks you 're weird? Will your brain view a news story on unemployment in your state as "When someone else does the same, there's no point in finding a better job? I'm not going to be good enough to beat out the rest.

Do you keep living the same life that you always have, because fear is preventing you from taking risks or making positive changes? How do you break your head's negative feedback loop? Try to replace positives with negative stories. If watching the television or reading sad stories on the internet triggers dread of those negative things that happen to you, stop taking that role. Spend your energy on feel-good success stories. The internet is loaded with good stories featuring an underdog accomplishing something great. Men battle for the good war. Stories that remind you of the world's good and the chance of positive happenings.

If fear of being laughed at keeps you from trying to take up yoga, read stories of people who, against challenges, have become yogi. If fear of rejection prevents you from asking that girl or guy out, read inspiring stories about couples that started in the circumstances similar to yours. If fear of messing up prevents you from trying, then that fear will hold you hostage. You have to choose to free yourself from that.

Have a realistic look to your worries. You 'd like to make a career change but you're too afraid to fill out work applications or submit your resume to prospective employers after seeing the television! Consider this: What's the worst possible thing to happen? Whenever you recognize that you're prevented from acting because of fear, ask yourself this question. What could be the wrong thing to happen? Type in your answers. Having anxiety in written form makes it harder for you to understand its irrationality.

Examples of Real Life include:

Fear: I want the job that I have seen posted, but they would not hire me anyway.

The worst possible result: you are filling out a work questionnaire and not receiving a response.

-- The worst case, you 're no worse off than you were before. The cost of your effort has been the time spent on applying.

Fear: I want my partner to do more work around the home, but if I ask them for assistance they may think I'm unable to.

The worst imaginable result: They grumble while cleaning the dishes for a few minutes.

-Best of all, they are not pleased to meet your offer, but they do so because marriage is a matter of partnership.

Fear: If I try a new haircut, it may look bad on me and people are going to stare. Worst possible result: You get a haircut you don't like.

-It's going to grow back out and you'll know that the particular look wasn't for you.

Fear: If I'm dining in a new restaurant I may not like the meal. The worst outcome possible: You've got a bad meal.

This should hardly prevent you from seizing a chance in the grand scheme of your life.

NOW those fears are unfounded as you can see. They 're not worth another moment of stressing or thinking what-if energy was wasted. Forget of the next possible scenario. Instead, think of the best result possible. Instead, keep that idea at the forefront of your mind. Remind yourself of the likelihood of a good outcome as much as possible. Note you can't control anything, including the future, but you control your actions and reactions.

Stop in her tracks, fearful worry. Deciding to seize the opportunity deliberately. Register for the job, and you're just as likely to get it as anyone else. Say what you need from your spouse and be grateful that they understand your position. Get the haircut because you will look amazing afterwards, because there is a good chance. Go to the restaurant to pick a new treat.

Agree you make mistakes sometimes. Much like you can't control every outcome, realize that any choice you make isn't going to be the right or the strongest. And this is fine. To be human is to err. Try watching the bigger picture. If you make an error, in an hour, a day, a week, a month, or a year later would you be angry about that? Odds are that next month, you won't even remember that mistake. You may have one or two regrets but are they stalking you like you thought they would?

You do know that a way to change your life is to train for results and that ultimately you can choose how to act in any particular situation. Fear is an emotion just like there is rage, happiness, disappointment and sorrow. You have control over how you feel. Mind the mantra, and choose faith over fear. Designed to be effective. Apply for the work you want and center your attention on how big a possibility could be.

When the client asks for an interview remind yourself that this will be a perfect time to reflect favorably on that question. For the interview pick the most flattering formal dress. Imagine the person you have ever seen with the most confidence and mimic their behaviour. Stand tall and hold your head high as you enter, offer a firm handshake and smile. Fake it, as the saying goes, until you make it. If you're behaving confident enough you'll start feeling genuinely confident.

When you think the anxiety is too big to surmount on your own, don't let yourself continue the emotional beatdown. Consider confiding about your fear with a friend or loved one in cases where you can talk through your fear without being obsessively concerned about it. Choose a dependable, rational, optimistic and frank mate. If someone with these qualities suggests your fear is irrational, then you are more likely to believe them.

Whenever possible, seek the factual information. With the introduction of the internet, at times we all fail to ask for expert advice. When we're not feeling well, there's a tendency to do a quick internet search to find out if medical treatment is needed. Choose any signs, check and 20 minutes later you'll be able to tell you that your days are numbered. Imagine you've got a friend who's telling you they have health concerns. The nature of their concern is to think they 're having a heart problem. Asking them what their doctor feels will be a rational answer. You ask them the issue, and they are told they haven't seen a doctor because they're scared of the answer.

This explanation illustrates how an overthinker has an influence on anxiety. The thoughts begin innocently enough and then they intensify into an unhealthy obsession.

-I'm not so good.

-I should probably go to the doctor.

-- Review my symptoms online.

-Read that the cause for the symptoms is very common.

-- Zero in on the least probable cause.

-- My grandpa was having this rare disease.

-What if I made it?

-Read that your demographic is uncommon for the disease.

-But of that, grandpa died.

-Read you should seek medical care.

-If I have this disease, I will be bankrupted by the operation, and then I will die anyway.

-If I get the illness, I need treatment.

-- That's what Grandpa died of and I'll go too.

-If I go to the doctor and they're finding something horribly wrong I can't work.

-If I can't work then I'm going to lose my career.

-If I lose my job I will not be able to afford medication.

– I'm going to die.

The fears spiraled out of control, just because you kept thinking about it. To the point you convinced yourself that death is imminent. How do you face your fear using the tools presented throughout this chapter? Identify the angst. I'm not feeling well and I'm afraid I might get very sick. Which might be the worst? I may just be really sick. Which is the best outcome? I have a common ailment that can be treated with ease. Decide to face the anxiety and arrange a rendezvous to see the psychiatrist. If you're afraid of the appointment, remember that you're more likely than not, it's going to be all right. Taking these steps to face your fear head-on will prevent hours, days or weeks of self-destructive overthinking and failure to tackle a problem. These instruments can be applied in any situation where fear paralyses. You just have to decide how to go about it. The word determine derives from the Latin word "determine," meaning cutting back. So, stand tall, be courageous and choose to cut off the other options. Choose a path and carry on. Focus on your goal, and plan to achieve it by losing sight of your fears.

Physically Stop the Cycle

The main focus at this point was to change your thoughts from cognitive distortions to more practical interpretations. In your goal, a shift in your thought habits is crucial to finishing over thought. Yet, it is not only instantly that the views shift. It will be a long process and you'll want to give in to your worried thoughts sometimes. You should make a adjustment to your daily behaviors to counteract the backsliding. Activities as boring as watching T.V. And browsing the internet leaves your intellectual energy too far free to think about. Shutting off an inquisitive mind on your thoughts can be as simple as "changing the channel." Pick something else to do. Something else. There's no way the brain would think hard of two things at once. Don't just sit in your head, playing your negative thoughts over and over. Act to have your attention turned elsewhere.

There will always be times when you can't stop with cognitive restructuring, list making, and setting a plan in motion. During such times, the actual breaking of the loop by action is beneficial. Constantly worrying trains your brain to think more about the preoccupation. Using other activities to distract your brain retrains it to stop the constant worry.

Physically demanding exercise is a great way to focus entirely on your worries, for a period of time that extends past when the exercise ends. Participate in an exercise that you like, such as competitive sport, fitness training, hiking, walking, etc. In general, you will soon find that you feel much more positive when you use pent-up energy for sports, rather than the obsessive overthinking in which you usually participate.

You concentrate your mind on the task of training, and look forward to a goal. The goal for your team can be a win, finish the class, or run or bike X number of miles. You've got feel-good endorphins entering the bloodstream by the end of the exercise and you feel better than ever, both emotionally and psychologically. When you feel that darn good it is hard to overthink. Most athletes use their run to clear their heads, running for as long as it takes to dissipate the bad emotions or anxiety. Others call the room the hole. We mentally force themselves into a state of mindlessness. That amount of physical exercise is not for everybody and I discuss it only as one of the many choices.

Research suggest that daily activity stimulates the brain specifically to increase the capacity of the prefrontal cortex and the temporal medial cortex. Those regions are the ones which control memory and thinking. Improving those particular portions of the brain can change your mind physically to stop the destructive overthinking. The relationship between the physical body and mind has a major effect on how you feel and think. It has been proven that maintaining this interaction strengthens the state of your emotions and how you communicate with the outside world.

There are secondary consequences of training, which help strengthen the ways of learning. Indirectly, completing a fitness goal serves to boost self-esteem and confidence. Trusty people with high self-esteem don't spend their time overthinking and worrying. Regular exercise helps improve sleep and reduce stress levels, both of which are the culprits in creating a ruminant environment. Any exercise will reap these rewards, so choose an activity you most enjoy. If you hate racing, do not become a driver. That will happen if you chose an action that you dread?

Very possibly, anything like this will come of it:

-Alarm is going off and your first thought is that you don't really feel like running.

-Shut the alarm off and go back to sleep.

-Wake up again, and regret your decision to sleep.

-- Sound like a loser when, on your drive, you see someone jogging out.

-Rinse and repeat the feelings of regret and failure until they escalate into "I will never be able to stick to running because I fail in everything I do" or some over-generalization of the kind.

Choose an activity that you can enjoy, or learn to enjoy. Singing, running, diving, gymnastics, kickboxing, zumba, singing, dancing ... it doesn't matter. Just exercise whenever you wish, in any way you like.

The best time to exercise is in two schools of thought: This is safe to start out early in the morning. The idea being that starting the day with a boost of feeling good endorphins creates momentum for the forward to carry the good feelings all day. The key to those who worry about first thing in the morning is to start with a clear mind. Individuals who tend to take advantage of early morning workout sessions because they have no time to come up with reasons to put it off. I heard people say they go to the gym until they're fully awake, but they don't change their minds.

Morning Workouts have advantages:

Consistency-Morning distraction like family reunions is less likely.

Convenience-First thing in the morning you can sleep in your exercise clothes and run straight out of the front door for a jog. If you're having trouble finding time for exercise this is a good method.

Domino effect-Making healthy morning decisions can encourage good day-round decision-making by "riding the high," if you like.

The second one is the end of the workday. These folks believe that physical activity at the end of the workday is effective in clearing the mind and eliminating the stress of that day to encourage a worry-free evening and putting an end to the day physically. PM practices also have the advantages of:

Accountability-Having a fitness partner for evening workouts is a lot better.

Stress Relief-Working out will clear your head at the end of a stressful day and avoid the inevitable loop of overthinking from taking over.

Endurance and power-Some people will work better later in the day after they are fully awake and have eaten a couple of times.

If procrastination is your problem, the way to go might be to practice morning workouts. If high stress levels after work triggers your unnecessary worry and anxiety, workouts in the evening are usually your best bet. In the end, the effect can only be felt if you do it, so choose the time that best fits into your life and be consistent. Take the physical leap to get your mind and ultimately your life better. Use physical activity to force obsessive thoughts out of your mind, and retrain your brain to improve your and others' interactions.

Your hobbies are ANOTHER TOOL IN YOUR ever-growing arsenal against overthinking. For example, reading requires far too much brain power to be worrying or focusing on your failures. You can read fiction, or you can get a double dose of nonfiction distraction. Learning something new encourages positive feelings by giving the sense of accomplishment to grasp a new concept or understanding that follows. If that happens to be your guilty pleasure, you could even read celebrity gossip magazines too. The material content isn't as important , as long as it positively affects your thinking.

Animals are distractions which are fluffy, feathery or scaly. Playing with dogs triggers feel-good hormones in your brain if you have them. A pet can be a fantastic distraction from too much worry and overthink. You'll both benefit from some reciprocal interaction. Some pets need just as much stimulation and exercise as you do. Taking your dog for a walk or park distracts you from worries and reinforces your dog bond for a double dose of feeling good. It's more entertaining to shine a laser pointer and watch your cat attack the wall than to replay a less than pleasant conversation with your mum. Look through your dog's eyes, take a long , hard look. He believes you are the world's best human being. Seek to see yourself through his eyes and iron out negative feelings. There's significant mental health advantages of owning a cat. Go out there, and play to enjoy the benefits for your furry pal.

When you don't have cats, try an animal shelter or a petting zoo. Try working at a shelter to help out other detractors who search for a daily dose of pet therapy. To do so offers many people a sense of purpose. Volunteering is a way of feeling positive for yourself and putting your life in context, of some sort. Changing your view of yourself, as discussed earlier, eliminates the desire to think over whatever shortcomings you believe you have. €Leaning litter, soup kitchen work, or community youth programs are all great options for spending your time and physical energy.

A good way to start is by searching the neighborhood calendar for entertaining distractions. Most towns have online event calendar. There are festivals with whatever is possible. It doesn't matter what concerns you. Jazz, pride, pumpkins, cranberries, trout, beer , wine, art, dogs, rabbits, cats, cucumbers, cars .... you name it, somewhere in the world there is a festival for that. Just wake up and go for a leisurely dose of entertainment. Holding and looking at the world's largest cucumber doesn't know how bad traffic this morning has been. In recent years communities are going beyond and beyond presenting entertainment opportunities. To distract yourself there are art shows, sporting events, concerts, and countless other activities. At a carnival, after all, it's hard to get upset. Positive energy is contagious at Community events. Cheering on your favorite team is so much more fun than sitting at home worrying about whether your boss thought your morning (three days ago) meeting comment was stupid. Get out there, and have fun. Enjoy the liberating feelings of happiness and carry them home with you. In the moments when worry threatens to take hold, reach for these fun memories. Use these opportunities to meet people who are positive, goal driven, to broaden your circle of positive influences.

You don't need to get overwhelmed by an exciting event. Just spend quality time with the ones that bring you joy. Playing games with friends, such as board games or interactive video games, is another positive way to occupy your mind. Spending time with the ones we care about improves our mental state. Such exercises should center your attention on constructive behavior that distracts you from your self-defeating worries. Positive interaction with those around you will enhance your relationships. We 're all responsible for creating our environment as discussed above. Your friends and family are responsible for their surroundings too. If your presence continues to bring positivity and positive feelings, you'll have more room in their lives. Nobody needs to hear you crying all the time. They have heard about your self-proclaimed, monumental disaster from five years ago and do not see it as such.

Pick up a relative or member of the family to talk. Don't get into the habit of conversing about your problems. Have a light-hearted chat. Concentrate on listening, rather than talking. Remember happy memories, and set new plans. Instead of the one in your head, focus on the conversation that you are having.

Go to your partner or spouse on a date. Make and obey a rule of "no worries." Spend a whole evening, or day, on fun activities and discuss other things than your usual concerns. A round of putt-putt, the arcade, or a movie are excellent distractions and conversational opportunities to use later.

If you want to sit alone at home, that's perfectly fine, just be sure to break the loop of pointless tasks that allow space to overthink. Do something which positively occupies your mind. Switch off the T.V. Series you've watched multiple times throughout, and choose a movie you haven't watched before. If you're extra persistent in overthinking, turn on a foreign film. At the same time, it is physically impossible to worry about and read the subtitles. If you need to play games on your phone, select those that are mentally stimulating, such as word puzzles or games for strategy.

It has been proved that listening to music clears the mind and encourages positive feelings. However, if you pick songs that dampen your spirits or have bad emotions associated with them, this approach will go horribly awry. Do not listen to the music you used to dance to, and your husband. This leads only to feelings of disappointment, a past that you can not alter and a future that you do not have. Instead, find music that you can't get upset while you listen. It might be the Jackson 5, for one person. Thinking negative thoughts whilst singing "ABC" at the top of your lungs would probably be physically impossible. "Shake it Off" maybe is a better choice than "She Hates Me."

Taking a minute to bring together a list of things you 'd like to pursue. And then continue to pursue one. When you do not find the exercise as calming as you would have thought, try another. Learning a new skill requires time , energy, and will help you stay away from your usual worry. The success of learning a new skill gives you a boost of confidence that can shadow negative perception of yourself. Accumulate some of these successes and you will be able to see yourself as almost an entirely new person of confidence.

Only playing music shows to have other benefits linked to quick thinking. Improving the way your brain works will make it possible to restructure your thoughts. Playing a musical instrument uses your brain differently from other activities, and thus exercises your brain differently. Some piano lessons benefit a lot more than just being able to play the piano. Replace piano with any decided instrument. Some examples of these benefits are:

-- Enhanced memory capabilities. Better recall means less worry about missing something.

-Team skills improved. Performing music with others requires outstanding competencies in coordination. Thinking as a team involves raising the inherent need for self-doubt and concern.

-Growing tolerance. Practicing a piece of music instills in you a knowledge which needs practice for performance. Practice needs persistence and knowledge before you excel, as you can fail several times.

There are many other hobbies which produce similar results. Knitting, drawing, learning a foreign language, creating templates and creative writing are popular choices. Any activity that engages both your hands and mind removes the ability to focus on worries or fears at the same time. Understanding any sport, including playing an instrument, requires the ability to lose and attempt again. Just drop a few stitches and try again, if you mess up. Carry those emotions through the rest of your life about failures, should you mistakenly buy the wrong wine for dinner, just sprint to the supermarket and try again. Any need to think for hours , days , weeks, months or even years on a minor mistake. Move into any hobby shop to find a diversion that suits your schedule, purpose, and level of ability.

Take the knowledge gained from this book to help choose an activity. The task that you want doesn't matter nearly as much as just completing one overall. Make a list of things you would love to do or go to. When you're not interested in music, do not listen to repeat "Shake it Off" as it was suggested by this article. If you'd rather go for a stroll, don't buy a bike. When you're allergic to cats, working at an animal shelter isn't a smart idea. The most critical thing to remember is does this practice have a good impact on you? It is counterproductive to select an activity which makes you feel sad, worried or anxious. If volunteering in a soup kitchen brings up bad memories of homelessness in childhood, please select another activity. Recognize that if an action is one of your own causes, you have power over whether you want to do it or not.

Set a time limit on picking the first task so you don't think too much about what you want to do the most. Two minutes is enough time to pick. Face your worry about failure and take the leap. If that is what appeals to you, decide to take the ukulele on. Make a choice then ask yourself, is the worst thing that could happen? If you sign up for a 6-week course on painting, just remember that the worst thing that can happen is, you 're not a fan. And that's all right, because there's no need to sign up again. That doesn't seem like spending hours mulling over a problem. Remember the possibly positive results. You 're perhaps going to love painting and find a new favorite hobby. You might get to meet some good people and make friends. Either way, painting a picture of a fruit bowl will be too busy for you to dwell on other past or future happenings. Keep in mind that you wouldn't have any more fun at home remembering how terrible you feel about this morning forgetting to feed the cat. Paint that fruit bowl and forget your mistake ... keep in mind that the cat forgot about it the moment you remembered and fed it. Find a way to set yourself free by forcing your brain to focus elsewhere if the "victim" doesn't remember the crime. There's endless list of physical activities for engaging your mind. Do new things, encounter new friends, build good memories and act and add fresh things to the mind to worry about. Find enjoyment in learning new skills. Learn from mistakes and build on successes. Find things at which you excel and use that information to replace repetitive thinking about your shortcomings. Do anything that lets you escape your own mind from the prison and use the experiences to build confidence and increase self-esteem. Learn to love the enhancement challenge and stop dwelling on every misstep.

Practice Mindfulness Daily

Previously, the use of a physical activity to overcome your destructive overthink and excessive worry has been discussed at great length. To fully break your overthinking habits, you need to change your mind. This chapter will focus on mental exercises that, with daily practice, will help you to transform your thinking and therefore your life using all the tips learned in this book.

The first step is an awareness of oneself. You've already made a lot of lists up here. You looked deep within yourself and wrote down your triggers, your cognitive distortions and their restructured counterparts, your anxieties, the hobbies you already enjoy and those you want to try. Through these exercises you have achieved a greater awareness of yourself. You have started to recognize what constant rumination does to you physically and mentally and admit that it makes you anxious, frightened, worried and tired. It's exhausting every day to criticise yourself. Remind yourself to return to the present when you feel vulnerable to a round of overthinking. Remember, your brain can not think about two things at once, so if you're focused on the present, it can't remember the past or worry about the future. Know in full that you can't influence the past or the future, no matter how much time you worry about them. Make it a priority to pull your mind squarely into the moment.

Treat yourself to gentlereminders all day long. If that is what it takes, hang up sticky notes all over your house and office. After a minor occurrence a simple "it doesn't matter" can end the snowballing of negative thoughts. Tell yourself consciously that if you don't think for tomorrow or next week, you don't have to waste money, or resources, looking after right now. Remain concentrated on the moment. Tell yourself tomorrow if you're really going to matter. If the answer is yes, this book needs to start anew ... All kidding aside, you probably won't care in the majority of situations tomorrow. Do not spend an unwanted disturbance on the moment. It stops you from enjoying your own life by destroying your time by dwelling on the past and imagining the future.

Practice thankfulness. Any situation could be worse, because the universe has people who struggle worse than you do. Within those claims, the conditions, no matter how dire, won't change the facts. Some of the most inspiring people ever suffered unimaginably, and maintained a positive outlook. Anne Frank comes to mind first. From her hiding place during World War II, written inside her diary pages that she believed people were good. If a Jewish person who is fleeing from the Nazi government can sustain a conviction that humans are intrinsically decent, perhaps everyone can see a positive side. We all know one person in our network seemingly happy all the time. You know that type of guy. You 're probably finding him irritating, and at least a little fictional. He always waves and salutes everyone he encounters with cheerfully. Ask him why this is so. More likely than not his answer will highlight the positive aspects of his life. This doesn't mean there aren't negative aspects, it means he has actively chosen to be thankful for the good.

For the many positive ones, much overthinking means keeping energy on the one negative moment. If the one negative moment uses hours of your time, think about how much time you can spend thinking about 100 positive moments. Make a list of all you need to be grateful for, and remember those things when the negativity strikes. Maybe you just thought you 'd buy a house at age 35, but here in your one-bedroom flat, you 're reading this. With every passing day, frustration rises up inside you. In your neighborhood, you see "For Sale" signs changing to "Sold." You swipe through photos of your friend's new houses on social media, and negative feelings all the time. The old one you'd spend hours remembering the money you spent on holiday a couple of years ago and how that might have been a down payment. Stop. Step back into the moment, and find something to be grateful for. Plenty of ideas come to mind:

- The apartment is controlled by temperature, so you're never cold in winter or hot in summer.

- They're not homeless. Situations are worse than yours.
- You've got all the great memories of that trip because it was one of your life's best weeks.
You still bump into the same man at the gym. He's more dominant than you and he's driving your dream car. The old you 'd succumb to envy, and make it sound meaningless. Jealousy is at the heart of much bad thought. Be aware of your negative thoughts, and turn them into thankful thoughts.
-You've noticed increased strength with his advice since you worked out together.
-Your current car is cheap to maintain, but it probably wouldn't be your dream car.

Practicing appreciation would take much self-consciousness, commitment and work. Your mind feels hard-wired to fret about and overthink obsessively. Taking a second to return to the present when you see the old patterns coming in, and consider a justification for being thankful. Create a new list of things that you would be thankful for regularly reminding yourself of all the positive things in your life. You will naturally notice the good in any situation with regular practice, instead of the bad.

No mention has yet been made of four full chapters in and meditation. What kind of guide is to stop overthinking? Meditation is the primary form of mindfulness meditation. A comparatively recent concept in the Western world, it has been used in east cultures to relax the mind for decades. This method is safe, and basically can be performed anywhere you can be. Meditation is an easy act but not an easy act. You've used the word but what does meditation really mean?

Merriam-Webster Dictionary describes the trance as:

'To participate in therapeutic activity (such as emphasis on one's breathing or mantra repetition) for the purpose of attaining an elevated degree of spiritual consciousness'

Every day do meditate with intention. The practice in the morning is easier, without filling your mind with all the conscious thought of the day. However, evening meditation has advantages. Like for physical training, try to train at a moment of greater value to you.

There are many different ways to meditate on the subject and a lot of experts. For a beginner, who is trying to rid their heads of excessive anxiety and overthinking, just concentrate on being conscious. Doing so is complex in its simplicity alone. Set a timer, no matter how much you want to train. Many experts recommend that beginners begin with 5 minutes and then add on if they wish. Place relaxed for you somewhere, and close your eyes. Concentrate on breathing. Use your nose to take deep breaths in and exhale through your mouth. Visualize a question when you inhale, and visualize it on the exhale flowing free. Continue this cycle until you have thrown aside all your worries. End the session without any of the problems that weigh you down. Take periods of conscious relaxation during the day whenever you find anxiety taking over.

Benefits of meditation:

-- Decreased gray matter after 8 weeks in the visual parts of the brain. A Harvard study links long-term meditation to the maintenance of gray matter, which decreases with age.

-Increases memory, improves decision taking.

-- Reduced stress, anxiety and depression.

Yoga is considered a physical exercise but for the meditative effects many individuals who practice it do so. Meditative yoga helps to calm an overactive mind, achieve true peace and affirm the relation between mind and body on a metaphysical basis. Unlike traditional meditation, meditative yoga starts by focusing your gaze at a particular place. You can look at a tree, a houseplant, a candle flame, whatever you think works for you. Direct your thoughts to something specific, like being in the present or breathing yourself. Keep that thought focussed. If your mind wanders, that is going to happen from time to time. Don't get mad about it, just let it reign down. The purpose of the practice is to learn to be present at any time and to refocus your mind, to free your headspace from negativity.

What are the Yoga benefits?

- Connection between mind and body improved. Encourages our desire to stay in the moment, and appreciation.

- Down with stress and anxiety.

If you're the type of person who doesn't handle silence well, meditation on mantra might be for you. This is a meditation that uses the chanting of a mantra as a way of freeing the mind and attaining awareness.

Whose benefits will chanting bring?

-- Destroy anxiety and depression. This is related to chemical reactions to stabilize the nervous response in the body.

-- Eliminates anxieties. Removing external objects and our bodies from attention restricts our capacity to think.

-- Sponsor love. It is believed that chanting would bring the practicer back to spiritual enlightenment. The meaning of this varies from person to person. Some people claim they are put on the same celestial plane as God through a chanting custom, while others claim it connects them to the world on a separate basis.

Like everything else we've discussed, the method you enact to practice mindfulness is personal preference. Try out any form that appeals to you, and reject the others. The form and length of practice is not as important as being done every day. Also, if you pick a technique and it doesn't work for you, then try another one over time. There are many ways to meditate, to chant and to do yoga. Try different types of things until you find personal success.

How else would you be conscious and present? Use your senses to the fullest. We've got five senses: taste, touch, scent, smell and vision. A mind full of worry mutes all those senses. Practice mindfulness by noting at any moment what your senses are gathering up. Stop, and smell the roses, as you have heard many times before.

Eating attentively after a meal will leave you feeling more satisfied. Turn off any distractions and focus on the platter. Look at the food, note the colorfulness of the vegetables. Smell the milk, what kind of herbs can you spot? And when you're taking a bite, taste the food almost absolutely. Take the little bites and deliberately chew them to savor the moment. As with meditative yoga, you focus on the item in front of you attentively.

Take note of how your muscles feel as they contract and release as you walk. Moving deliberately involves making care of how you feel when you pass. Pay attention to your pace, and feel each step hitting your foot. Staying in the moment even as you are walking through a crowded room. Let any move intentional, instead of just running through the motions.

Sense the breath. Inhale, and deliberately exhale. Seek finding it when you look at it, really. Beware of shades and angles. Listen to the discussion in full. Hear the words that you are speaking and the ones that you are being told. Taking in every word on the website as you type. Ear the texture of the vestments.

Use all these tools to live in the present securely rooted will free you from anxiety. I'm going to say again; he can't worry about a busy mind. Since idle hands are playing ground for the Devil, an idle mind is vulnerable to obsessive thoughts. Keep your mind listening closely to stave off your own negativity. The essence of living your life is the daily practice of mindfulness. Having exist inside the walls of one's own head isn't even alive. Drop pessimistic feelings realizing that, in your case, you are not a mere spectator. You and you can only decide how to react to any situation, including whether to act on your thoughts or not.

Studies have shown that a habit requires 21 days to form. Continuous mindfulness practice will change your life in this short span of time.

Apply the changes outlined inside this book to your mind and body. Hold your head firmly rooted in the moment and stop disruptive overthinking and unnecessary anxiety, stop procrastinating and start getting the results you are hoping for.

Prepare For Success

Some of the most critical considerations that will decide how the day would continue may be how you start the day. Hectic mornings tend to get hectic afternoons etc. An effective tool for ending overthinking is to avoid it happening. Do you know the breakfast is mostly missed because you waste so much time choosing what to wear? Will lack of coordination preclude you from performing a big task? Will you still intend on having something done tomorrow? Last Luncheon? The month's First? How is life getting simpler? When is the time? As the start date becomes increasingly vague, it will very likely never happen.

When such conditions sound familiar, action should be taken to break the loop. And as the saying goes, "dress for the role you desire instead of the one you've got," you have to plan for the future you desire, rather than the one you have.

Take a moment to think about the way you start every day. Will you find your daily routine becoming a day to day frustrating occurrence? Have you ever abandoned projects, so you don't know where to start? Do you feel trapped in a constant failure loop, and do you no longer see the point of trying something better? Will you go to bed only to lay awake at night and ask where the day went wrong? Are you focusing on one mistake you made a decade ago that might cause your current failure in some way?

The over-thinker considers these forms of negative feedback loops normal. Rumination is our tendency to avoid worrying about our mistakes / failures. Luckily there are basic improvements which can interrupt the loop when done regularly.

Spend a few extra minutes each night to make sure they get off to a good start the next morning. Think of it as setting up yourself to succeed. Recall the 5 Ps: Proper Preparedness Prevents Poor Performance. Doesn't the title of this book directly contradict your thinking about tomorrow? You shouldn't be living in this moment? The difference between destructive overthinking and performance preparation is that one ends up with a solution. Worrying for worries offers no solution to the issue.

This can quickly escalate to self-doubt related stress for the overthinker and result in the task going on another day without completion. Strengthening, then, what your worrying mind suggested. With each smaller portion of the task accomplished, you reinforced the idea that you can succeed. Every tiny moment of success creates faith that you can do what you need to do.

If the thought of breaking your "cold turkey" routines is too overwhelming, you can choose to arrange a fixed amount of time for contemplation into your day. It is appropriate as long as you try to hang on to a fair period of time. No more than 20 minutes a day will be committed to thinking on time. Set a timer, and just let yourself think about anything you want. Consider every result of a situation, ruminate on things you wish you could change, and so on, until the timer rings back. Then you have to stop straight away and go back to something more productive. You won't need the daily rumination any more over time. Without the desire to waste that time on negative thoughts the set time will come and go. Only stop fitting it into the day when the time comes.

CONCLUSION

Thank you for reading this book through to the end. Let's hope it's been informative and able to give you all the tools you need to reach your goals whatever they may be.

The next step is to reaffirm that you are on your way to becoming a better, fuller person every day. Review how far you have gone, and be proud! As with anything, consistency and determination are key to success. Believe in yourself and your willingness to make the requisite improvements to achieve your goals. If you've eliminated the noise from your head, each and every day you convert overthinking into concentrated achievement. You may have heard "easier said than done" many times over. Well, you should be excited to learn how to do what you set your mind to do. For a long time you had wanted to make a change. Taking the move toward reaching your goals is something that other will cannot do.

It is times like this, after taking a big step forward in my life, when I start to think about how far I have come. Sometimes it is difficult to appreciate your progress when you are in the heat of battle and struggle every day during the beginning, middle, or even close to the end of your efforts. There's nothing better than walking up onto the final rung and looking down in your wake to see all the moves done.

Remember when you sat at square one, unable to free yourself from the overthinking chains? I know that well — I was there myself. To get up and say, I'm ready to make a transition, takes a lot of confidence. This saddens me to know that, in their whole lives, many people tend to overthink and over-analyze, ignoring the insights and understanding a rational mind can understand. It's easy to slip into the comfortable habits of mindless eating, checking every few minutes for a phone or tablet, and going to bed later and later until your system is out of sorts. Sometimes, giving in seems too easy, and letting what is easy overshadow what's worth working for. You don't need to be a slave to overthink, and maybe you can take what you've learned and help change lives around you.

Maybe you know someone who seems to be struggling to overthink, develop a tough mind, stress the daily challenges and stress just like you were at the beginning of your journey. Think of reaching out and sharing what you have learned. Nothing is stronger than exchanging your experiences with someone who can use it to make the meaningful improvements in themselves that you have seen happen. Maybe he's a colleague, a spouse or a close friend. Many people from different walks of life will benefit from this book's changes, so why not share your story!

Keep in mind that overthinking is a habit that has taken time to develop, as such it will also take time to replace those habits with new ones. To make the change, it will take daily application of the methods you choose to implement. Over time, consciously changing how you thought can avoid the damaging overthinking, procrastination, and unnecessary stress to strengthen your and others partnership. Refer to the chapters to maintain the personal changes as needed in the future.

9 781802 100785